Strokus

A Journey Through Stroke and Recovery

This is my story about the struggle to regain normalcy after a stroke.

Sharon Watt

Strokus

Dedication

This book is dedicated to Mom,Dad,Jess,
Beverly and all of the Angels in Scrubs at
Christiana Care that helped me along the road
to recovery, as well as my friends and family
that visited and encouraged often.
"Thank you" just isn't enough to express my
gratitude!

Table of Contents

1.

INTRODUCTION

I have always been exceptionally motivated and active, especially with tasks around the house. I love renovation projects, painting and so many other things. So the massive hemorrhagic stroke took me completely off guard on that cold February night of President's Day. I had been hard at work ripping up the carpet in my bedroom.

It started with a headache that made me very tired and I fell asleep laying on the rolled up carpet that had yet to be taken out to the trash. I had been texting with my daughter's, who was at college in Tennessee. I laid my cell phone on the dresser that had been moved to the center of the room and I fell asleep fast and soundly and awoke to vomiting. I tried to get up, but i was not able to. My hair was soaked with vomit. I called my dogs into the room with hopes that they would be able to help. They were more concerned about getting their heads rubbed and kissing my face than getting me up.My cell phone had been ringing and pinging, but it was too far away to reach so I went back to sleep. When I awoke again, the sun was coming into my room and i heard someone come in the front door. The dogs were barking.

Mom had come over to check on me along with my two of my coworkers. My boss called my mom when I didn't show up or call in at work. They tried to get me up but then they realized that I didn't have use of my left side and they called the EMS. When the ambulance arrived, my blood pressure was over 200 over 100 and my speech was slurred, so they rushed me to the hospital. I don't really remember the ambulance ride, what happed in the ER, or what they said to me. I think I slept through most of the shuffling and tests. I remember that I was in at least 3 different rooms in the hospital and my sister drove in from Ohio, flew my daughter in from college in Tennessee and picked her up at the airport on her way to the hospital It was great to have them both home to help mom and dad with my dogs and keep up with all of my movements in the hospital.ICU, step down and then a regular acute care room. After a week of bouncing around the Christiana Hospital,I was moved to the Wilmington Hospital for the long road of rehabilitation. I knew that facility very well because my dad had spent several months there over the past few years. My parents had become friends with one of the aids and her husband so we knew that they would take good care of me.

2.

MY BRAIN HURTS

Stroke recovery is a long process and is different for everyone. For me, the stroke was in the right side of the brain, so my left side was affected. I couldn't walk, stand, or do anything with my left hand. It created a frustration like i had never had before. I couldn't do the things that had always been so easy and natural PS (pre-stroke).

There are a linty of things that health care professionals use to mark the severity of a stroke and the same tasks and questions are repeated multiple times each day and every time you see someone new.

What day is it?

What is the date?

Who is the president?

Blink your eyes.

Stick out your tongue.

SMILE!...... *Stop saying that to women already!!!!!*

Squeeze my fingers...... *but i can't... how frustrating!*

Touch your nose.

Repeat what I just said....... *OMG stop giving me number sequences to remember!*

Does anything hurt?... *Yes, my brain!!*

I slept with ice on my head for weeks. It was like a teddy bear for my brain. It was cool and soothing and allowed me to shut down at night. The nurses and aids at both hospitals all learned quickly that I wanted two ice packs at night. One for my shoulder and one for my head.

3.

FAMILY FIRST

I have a daughter, Jess. She was attending college over 12 hours away, in Tennessee. Following my stroke, my sister, Beverly, quickly made the decision to fly her home and her amazing neighbor made the flight arrangements while she was driving. It was very generous and definitely needed. Jess' always positive outlook, encouragement and rationale are hard to duplicate and are exceptionally useful. While she was home, she made the decisions that I could not. She, along with my mother and sister, talked to the doctors and kept track of what was happening. She was, and still is, a Godsend. She stayed long hours and helped me with everything from texting my friends to getting Wawa smoothies for me every day. She was the equivalent to an information officer. She and my sister made sure that they took information in and gave it out as needed via text, phone, and Facebook. She also understood my limits and was able to break things down to a level that I could comprehend. She is still explaining what happened in the first few days to me when I forget.

I cried at the sight of my daughter and sister on that first night. I was awestruck that they had made the trip when they had very full and busy lives out of state. My sister is a swimming coach with several teams in Ohio and it was finals season. My daughter had only been back to school for a couple of weeks and was very stressed out about an incident that led to some unexpected legal repercussions.

Before the stroke hit, I had been texting with my daughter. Apparently, our last text exchange consisted of her telling me to go to bed and me saying, "Who needs sleep?" Yes!, That sounds like me!

My first night in the hospital, I could not do anything alone and was under near constant supervision and evaluation. My mom and sister helped me eat, nurses kept me monitored and aids did the rest. My daughter kept me entertained and helped me with some of the things that only she understood, like putting my hair up and making sure I could use my bed controls, iPad, etc. My care was definitely a team effort!

My sister let my friends and extended family know what was happening through Facebook posts and the people at work called her and my mom for updates regularly. My daughter, had the task of notifying my special friends via my phone. Both were instrumental in making sure I felt connected to the people that mattered most to me. I will forever be grateful to them for that and so much more!

Being the official Next of Kin and Decision Maker for your lone parent at 19 is a hard task. I think at times, it may have hurt my mother's a feelings a little, but I wanted Jess to be the one to gather information from the medical team. I knew that she would know exactly what I needed and wanted. She knew how to stand up for me and wasn't afraid to do it, just as she saw me do hundreds of times with my parents when they were in the hospital and she was drug along for visits.

I recently learned that Jess even sat with me through my initial angiogram (which I'm sure was not easy)and spoke with all of the doctors during my first week in the hospital. She retained the information and now explains it to me as I need or ask for it. When she was able to go, she attended follow up doctors appointments with me. It was nice that the doctors and she remembered each other and she patiently explains things that happened during the blank time to me.

In addition to all of the shit going on with me, Jess had her own holy hell happening in Tennessee, where she had been accused of an assault, told by the college staff that they thought she was lying when she told them her version of the incident and then she was brought up on charges. This all happened around the time of my stroke and she now blames herself for causing my blood pressure and stress level to rise and cause the stroke, which couldn't be further from the truth, but the thought is so anguishing to her and her anguish is very painful for me.

Looking back, gives me an even greater appreciation for her maturity especially when I add in the fact that her mom, the only parent she really knows, almost died and she still kept it together like the champ that she is and went back to school and managed to pull through on the Dean's List!

While I was incapacitated, Beverly really stepped in and helped her by finding a lawyer, and getting to the nitty gritty of what was happening. It was such a relief to not have to deal with that while in the hospital. The lawyer was very nice to Jess and Bev and told them that he would take care of everything for her.

Following the stroke, my parents took my dogs to their house to take care of them for me. At the time, there were five, whom their neighbors despise and call the police about whenever they are dog sitting. It's a big mess, but they did it and my sister was a huge help with them; sometimes taking them out to potty on leashes so she could control their barking.

The dogs were upset. They saw the whole thing, from working on the carpet to not being able to get up, to strangers and grandma at the house taking me away. There was no way to explain it to them, so they would sniff my clothes when Mom took them home to wash them. That was there only confirmation that I even still existed.

Jess being home and seeing them regularly that first week certainly helped calm them and ease them into what was their new norm for a few weeks.

Not having the dogs around was hard for me. Although none are Emotional Support Animals, anyone with animals knows that they are all emotional support animals. For me, Zenith, the Samoyed mix was like my soul mate. He seemed empathic. He could feel my pain, joy, frustration, etc. and was always by my side. He was my heart and soul. My forever dog! He was old and I worried about him.

Twelve years old was up there for the breed and I
knew that every day was a blessing to have him. I
missed him and the others immensely. Bev and Mom
sent me pictures and FaceTimed with me regularly, so
I could see them and know what they were doing.
Who knows if they recognize me when I talked to
them, but it made me feel better..... a bit less like I
was abandoning them.

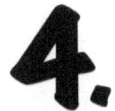

VISITORS

I cannot say enough good things about all of the people that came to visit me and especially those that brought me treats like smoothies from Wawa, non-hospital dinners, and cookies for my nightly sweet dreams snacks.also Pat and Joe for making home cooked meals for my parents and sister several times during the course of my hospital stay and when I was recovering at Mom and Dad's house.

Of course the notifications by Bev and Jess led to so many things, including questions, visitors, and lots of well wishes. The first visitors after my family were very best friends, Ron and Bill. I woke up from a nap and they were standing in the doorway. They are amazing men and are great huggers. I felt stronger with them there.

I had a lot of visitors from work. Almost daily, someone that worked with me stopped in. They were great about bringing me news from the office, but not stress or drama and I greatly appreciate that. They also honored what they knew to be my wishes with regard to the events that I plan. My associates and I all appreciate that. They also did not just replace me with someone else, they split up the tasks and tackled them one by one. They also kept the news of my stroke very quiet and did not tell people outside of the organization or my circle of friends.

The folks from my department came in regularly to visit me. Usually two or three at a time and often with homemade cookies(the only thing other than Wawa smoothies that I had requested). One day when they came in, they shared some videos with me that they had taken of each department around the City municipal building, where I work.

Someone from work even took the initiative to go to each department and record a get well soon or best wishes video for me. They brought them in and airdropped them all to my phone so I could keep them. The videos were digital Get Well Soon cards and I loved them! It was very thoughtful, as were the visits from other city employees throughout my hospital stays.

My cousin's wife compiled a package of get well cards from my dad's side of the family and sent them to me. My sister helped my open and go through them. It was very kind and greatly appreciated.

According to my friend, John, I am Superwoman! So, he brought me superwoman socks and sunglasses, which I wore with pride throughout my time in PT and when they had bright lights shining in my eyes for exams. Thank you to John for seeing my strength when I felt weak and for being a cheerleader for my recovery. John will find his way back in the story when I ramble on about the puppies!

5.

CAN I PLEASE JUST PEE ALONE?

Being in a hospital long-term has it's downfalls. There are endless precautions and restrictions, of which, I cannot name them all. After a stroke, the two most annoying for me were being restricted to a wheelchair and not being allowed to do anything alone, including pee.

In the beginning, the staff was obsessed with making me try to use a bed pan. *No, Thank you! I'm 48, not 84!*

After the bed pan, they wanted to strip me down and put me on a lift with my ass hanging out to put me on a commode in the middle of the room. Both are extremely humiliating experiences! Somehow the staff forget that even though you had a stroke, you do still have feelings that can and are bruised by a lack of compassion and thoughtfulness. You still want and need modesty to be a thought and for your desire for it to be considered.

Someone would literally stand in front of me and watch, then measure or analyze and record my productivity in the restroom. It was like nurses do to babies when they are first born, except the urine was scrutinized as much as the feces. What color was it? Did it have an odor? Was it cloudy? How much was there? No pressure! If you have bathroom shyness, having a stroke will not be easy for you. If, however, you are all about public urination, here's your chance to shine!

6.

STROKUS

Strokus is a word that I created during my time in the rehab unit of the hospital. I define it as the inability to focus because of a stroke. Distractions are amplified and you get sucked into them easily. I would say."squirrel" to my therapists when I got distracted by something (taken from the Disney movie, "UP") It was a joke at first, but quickly caught on as a way for me (and the therapists) to know when I was distracted by a person or activity taking place nearby.I still hear the "squirrel" reference in my head every time I am in the car with my mom. As she points out all of the things on the side of the road, I hear it and realize how distracted she and so many other people are in the world everyday... even people that didn't suffer from a stroke. There're are so many squirrels... recognizing them is a key to becoming more self-aware (which is important during stroke recovery).The word, strokus has now evolved for me and is about the focus needed to recover from a stroke. It's all about visualizing goals and focusing on one task at a time. Master one goal or task then move on to the next task or goal.Setting goals after a stroke can give both you and your therapists something to work toward. Some will be set by the therapists' regular protocol and others, you will need to set for yourself.My biggest goals were:-

Walking-

Putting a ponytail in my hair-

Smiling-

Living independently-

Driving-

Going back to work

some of these goals, I have accomplished and some, I have not, but continue to work on. As with all things in life, goal are ever changing and evolving

PS 3 months, my goals were:

- Mastering the ponytail.
- Going back to work.
- Going to amusement parks.
- Walking a mile or more each day

- Some I mastered easily and others have proven to be a challenge.

Now, PS over a year, my goals are:
- Not having knee and leg pain.
- Being able to exercise regularly, including mushing with the dogs.
- Tackling home improvement projects without fear.
- Finishing and publishing several books.
- Spending days at Hersheypark and tackling the hills there with ease.
- Walking in heels without a cane.
- Not living in fear of another stroke.

7.

I MISSED THE BOAT

It's no secret, in my circle of friends and family, that Train is my favorite musical group. The lead singer, Pat Monahan and I have very similar taste in music. So, I very much enjoy listening to his show on SirusXM, called Train Tracks and think that's one day, my daughter , Jess will be on the show! I often hear a song once and tell Jess that it will be a hit (or not). Her style fits right in and it may just be a chance for her to be heard one day.

Anyway, The group has been holding music cruises called, Sail Across The Sun for several years. I wanted to go from the start, but couldn't pull it off for various reasons, but in the summer 2017, I made the decision that I would go on the 2018 cruise, so I finally booked the cruise in the summer prior to my stroke. It was a dream come true and Jess and I were so excited! Around Christmas, theme nights were announced and I went crazy buying costume accessories, flair, and fabric to create some masterpieces. When I got home from my birthday trip to Disney and Jess was a back at school in Tennessee, I started working on mermaid jeans, Madi gras tops and glow-in-the-dark sneakers.

Little did I know that I would never use these items, because there was no way that the doctors, therapists, and my family were going to let me go and Jess was not going to go without me. She knew how much I wanted to go and said that the trip was for me, not her, so either we both went or no one did. I was crushed! Heartbroken! Why did I live through the stroke, if I couldn't spend time enjoying life and bringing joy to my daughter?

The cruise was during Jess' spring break. So rather than enjoying ourselves on the ship, Jess spent her break at the hospital, helping and encouraging me to get better and I felt guilty about ruining her break. I laid in the hospital at nights during the cruise and I would watch videos that were posted from the cruise and Jess brought one of my Train concert T-shirts to wear during physical therapy. Sometimes, I would put my headset on and listen to a playlist and I cried every time Drops of Jupiter played. Sometimes, I still do. I was so angry about the stroke and even more so about missing the cruise. Thank God for travel insurance and to Sixthman, the cruise coordinators, that sent me a patch and a mug from the cruise. It was a beacon of joy in a sea of sadness.

The days were long for me that week. Missing not only the cruise, but also a visit to Graceland and visiting friends in NOLA prior to the cruise that had been planned as part of our fun music week.

I don't think that anyone but Jess knew how truly devastated I was. My sister sort of chuckled when I mentioned the cruise right after the stroke. I can remember her laughing and saying, "pfffff! You're not going on that! I hope you have travel insurance. I'll call and cancel it!" What?! No way! I have waited for five years for this! How could it be ruined so quickly? I made plans. I'm going! But regardless of how much I wanted to do it, the doctors and staff also agreed that it was too much and too soon.

So, I longed fir the sunshine to come in the window and to hear a Train song in the Gym, so I could imagine the fun of being there ... just not Drops of Jupiter, please!

Today, the line up for SATS6 was announced and, just like two years ago, I am determined to go. It's always a financial challenge to do big trips like this, but I have worked hard to get to where I am today and I am determined to go. The dates for the next trip are one month after my 50th birthday until the two year anniversary of the stroke. Jess will turn 21 in October. So, we will celebrate on the 2020 SATS cruise. We will celebrate life and success and progress. We will celebrate our birthday milestones, her impending college graduation, and the joys of life and music... something that we have always enjoyed together, from her first concert (Eddie Money) at 3 months old to our last concerts together in September (Elton John and Niall Horne). We have traveled to DC, NYC,

Hersheypark, and more, chasing bands and screaming the words that are part of our spirits. we have seen Train together at least eight times over the years and we are looking forward to seeing them again this summer in Camden, NJ.

We have also seen many of the groups that were part of SATS past and wish we could see them all again on the next cruise. From Rachel Platten in Philly who spent some time sitting with us for a bit at he HardRock Cafe to seeing Andy Grammer at the Wilmington Flower Market, Matt Nathanson with Train one year at Hersheypark. These are the people and sounds that fill our hearts and fuel our spirits. They also help to fuel Jess' drive to be a producer and audio tech. I am so proud! She's a great singer/songwriter with an amazing ear and one day, she will be the creator of amazing music that others like us, will appreciate deeply.

I'm excited about the addition of the Rembrandt's being part of the SATS6 cruise, because their most popular song, will speak of our story, I'll Be There For

You, as I am for her and she for me. I promise that I will cry during Don't Grow Up So Fast again, like I always do when I look at her during the song.

This topic drained me when I talked about it during psychotherapy a few weeks ago and will probably drain me for a few more days now that it's been written, read, and reread. Because I have PTSD about the stroke, I live in fear of having another one, about losing abilities that I worked so hard to regain, and about missing out on the everyday joys of life, like SATS6. So everyday until the cruise, I will wonder if I will actually be able to go this time. I don't want to book my hotel too early or my daughter's flight. I don't want my hopes to be so high that I have a chance to be sucked into the misery that I was last year, when I couldn't go. I doubt there will be much effort put into flair or costumes this time, because I don't want to build myself up like that again. My devil horns(that were just like Pat's) sit on a shelf in my room and are a reminder that I didn't get to stand on the deck that night with all of the other little SATS5 devils in red and angels in blue jeans.

8.

THERAPY

Post-stroke therapy begins in the minutes following your stroke and never truly ends. Once you realize that there are things that you are not able to do, your therapy has begun. It starts out as memories, recollections, and desires. About a week after my stroke, i moved from acute care to rehab and the real work began. There, I was put on a schedule of therapy five times per day(2 sessions of both physical and occupational and 1 speech).in order to clarify, I'd like to explain a bit about what each therapist focused on during out sessions.

Physical therapy - Worked on large muscles and balance, walking, transferring from the wheelchair to other places.

Occupational therapy - Worked on arms and fine muscle movement. Hand and finger coordination and strength

Speech therapy - Focused on visual and mental acuteness as well as building facial muscles, that included speech and communication skills and memory.

I loved my therapists! Sarah, Jenna, Annie, Dani, Phil and all of the other therapists, nurses, doctors, and aides were hard working angels in scrubs. They let me know, despite their efforts to keep my ass in a wheelchair, that recovery is possible, but not easy. They taught me how to do a lot while I was in the rehab center and prepared me to go home to a more independent, but still supervised life.

Because my stroke was in the BasilGanglia section of the brain, everyone used the term, "impulsive" with me. The area is an impulse center so its a standard thing, but it didn't make it any easier to hear and it made my skin crawl every time I would hear someone say that I could not be left unsupervised because I was impulsive...*just shut the hell up and don't say things like that in front of me or other patients.* It's rude and not necessary unless someone has done something to deserve the label or treatment. Hearing things like that make you think that you have done something wrong even when you have not. It made me shut down some days because of frustration.

Don't get me wrong, I would participate and do what they asked on those days, but I was not my chatty or happy self. I was only going to do what I was told and nothing more on those days, because I knew that if I did, it would be blamed on my "impulsiveness". *That's right, give my family and co-workers more words to use as swords against me!* That is exactly what I need! Don't let Sharon make a decision, she is too "impulsive" and won't make a good decision.

This was especially true as the time neared for me to be discharged and I needed things in order to go home, like a transport wheelchair, a bed on the 1st floor, clothes that I could dress myself in, etc. I was so happy to have Amazon, Groupon, Wayfair, and an iPad. I bought my own transport wheelchair. I got a day bed for the living room. I got clothes that I could put on and off by myself. And, I was called "impulsive" at least a hundred times for it! I saw it as taking care of myself the only way that I could, but to my mom and my sister, I was being impulsive and careless with my spending. They were trying to bring me clothes and shoes for therapy, etc, but couldn't find some of the things that I asked for, so they went to Walmart and bought me shoes that were a size too big(so it would be easier to get my feet into them never mind tripping over the extra space) and other things that I didn't really need, but they thought that I did.

I appreciate that they cared enough to try, but asking me would have been appreciated even more. Ask Questions like the ones below, rather than assuming you know what's best.

"What do you think you will need when you go home?"

"What are your concerns?"

"What are you looking forward to?"

"What do you think your biggest challenges will be?"

Do you have clothes and shoes that you can manage yourself right is there something that we should look for or get you?"

"Do you have a favorite pillow or blanket that you would like to sleep with?"

Since I was not going to my house first, these questions would have been even more relevant. Going back to the comfort topic a few chapters ago, make sure people are not just providing the basic necessities, but also, the homey comforts; Manicures, hair color and cuts, massages, essential oils, warm socks, etc.

I'm going to talk about rehab in general now, because it wasn't just my experience as a patient, but also as a family member dealing with my dad's rehabilitation multiple times.

Caring for one's health and personal hygiene is not always something that the patient can just do on his or her own. Sometimes a little (or a lot) of help goes a long way. Shaving is much more challenging when you are not allowed to shower yourself....and I'm just talking face and legs right now, so you can just imagine how difficult the more tender areas are. You are not given a razor, so families, that is something important to buy or get for the patient. When you are used to shaving your arm pits daily, a week or two's growth feels disgusting! Regardless of how much deodorant you use, it never feels dry. Which leads me to mention that you should be asking for the brand of deodorant to get the patient and not just picking up the sale or dollar store variety. It will not be the same and the goal should be to provide the patient with an experience as close to their pre-stroke life as you can. If the extended family gathers for Sunday dinners, take the dinners to the patient for a few weeks. They still want to belong and keep as much of their PS routine as they can.

I can say that I honestly believe that I had many more comforts than most stroke patents because I was not shy about asking for things, like smoothies, cookies and milk, etc. People pulled through because I asked in many instances. It wasn't easy to ask, but after people asked every day, I had time to contemplate it and was prepared the next time someone asked. "I'm going to come back to visit next week, is there anything you want or need?"

"A Wawa smoothie would be amazing, thanks!"

One of my friends that lives in Nevada, even mailed cookies for me. So sweet!

Strokus

Thank you to everyone that tried to keep me
comfortable!

9.

ALMOST HOME

Home

After 6 weeks of in-patient therapy, I was released into my parents' care and in-home therapy was arranged.

Mom drove me home from the hospital and my wheelchair came with us. So, out of the car and into the wheelchair, I went. My sister and MOm then took me to the backyard to see the dogs. We were so happy to see each other, it made me cry. I was finally with my fur babies again. They all ran over to greet me, but were a little shy about the wheelchair. Not to worry, I won't be using this for long. When I got out of it

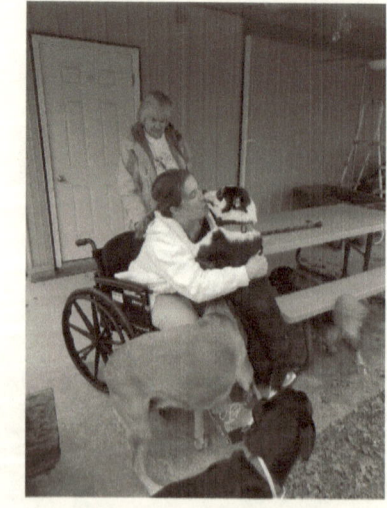

to go up the steps, that was my last time using it. It sat in a corner of the room until I moved home and then it moved to their porch.

It's never easy to move back into your parents' house as an adult... and that is especially true when your parents and your big sister want to treat you like a child again. Though I must say that I did enjoy waking up to the smell of breakfast being cooked some days.

While my sister was still home, she and mom moved my old bed from the second floor into the living room, so I wouldn't have to navigate the stairs. They got clothes that they thought I would be able to change into and out of easily from my house, and really did a lot to try to make it comfortable for me.

The best thing was that it was Easter weekend when I was released, so my daughter came home from college to visit and help out.

Jess is, by far my biggest advocate and motivator. In circumstances when I was frustrated and not able to do something, Mom would do it for me, but not Jess. Nope, she would yell like a drill sergeant at me until I was successful at doing it myself. She knows exactly when to push me and make me work harder and when I have had enough. She's not afraid to let other people know when they need to back off too. She is absolutely amazing! One minute she might be yelling for me to open the bottle myself and the next she's telling me that I look tired any maybe need to rest for a while.

I was working on getting my fingers to function better while I was in therapy, so when we were FaceTiming, she would say things to irritate me, so I would give her the middle finger. If I used my right hand, she would laugh and say ,"Now let's see you do that with the other hand!" So I would and she would tell me that was better. It's insane how hard I worked just to give my kid the finger! ...and she knew it was with love!

At my parent's house, I had in home therapy. Mike was my primary provider for PT and an Occupational Therapist came out to work with me a couple of times, but released me afterI had about 10 days. Mike was with me three times each week for several weeks. We started where I left off in the hospital and I was walking without the hemi cane in no time. I did a lot of work in between our sessions and got outside as much as I could. Mom and Dad have a nice cement area outside of their house, where I would go to practice side steps, marching, and walking backwards. When Mike would come, he could tell that I practiced, so we started venturing out farther and farther. It was hard, but I was doing it! I was sent home with a wheelchair and did not touch it beyond the first day. I did use the hemi cane a lot in the beginning, but moved away from that fairly fast, too.

This was truly a case of mind over matter... I set goals regularly and didn't give up until I achieved them. Little things like opening a water bottle felt like I had conquered Mt Everest. These goals were not set by my therapists, but by me. If I failed when I attempted something, it often became a new goal. Tying my shoes, taking the dog out on a leash, cooking dinner, getting into the bathtub for a bath, washing my own hair, pulling my pants up, zipping a jacket, and buttoning a button. They seem like easy tasks, but I had to re-learn all of them and had to work to do it.

10.

The Z Dogs!

My dogs were still at my parents' so I got to sleep with them and got lots of the love that I missed out on when I was in the hospital. I had 5 dogs; Zadie, Zoliver, Zara, Zenith, and Zoya. They are all mixes and are my recreational dogsled team. We have spent years together and they provide great comfort to me. I know that they missed me as much as I missed them. So it was wonderful to be together again.

Of course, nothing in my life is that simple and I found out that two of mom and dad's neighbors were harassing them about my dogs being there. So they were trying different methods to keep them from barking, limiting their time outside, and even restricting them to a leash to go out. Even though I was home, they were still the ones caring for them and I was the cuddlier. Zoya, Zenith, and Zadie could not get enough love some days and would jump in bed for snuggles regularly.

With me home, one of the challenges was to put the dogs away in another room while the therapists were there. They didn't like it, but did it anyway.

11.

Home Sweet Home!

Going to my own house was a huge step! Mom and I went to my house several days before I was allowed to go home to work on getting it ready. Mom helped me get the daybed set up and we took what I needed to my house. So, once Mike released me from in-home PT, I was ready to go home and start outpatient PT. I had driven a couple of times while I was at mom's, much to her dismay. So, when I was ready to go home, I was ready to be independent. I packed my stuff and we put it in Mom's car, then I told the dogs to get in the car (my car). Most of them jumped right in, but had to help Zenith, the old man that was also my dearest love. He

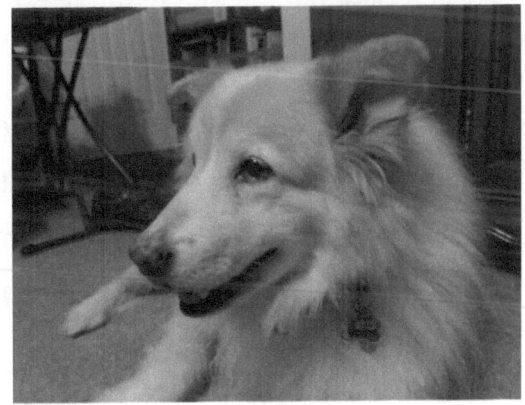

couldn't climb onto the passenger seat, so he curled up on the floor of the front seat and I closed the door. He smiled.

Once we got home, I took the younger dogs in then went back to get Zenith. I opened the door and he rolled out and onto his feet. He walked with me around the car and up the driveway and onto the porch. He was slow, like me, but he did it. We walked to the door. He collapsed when he crossed he threshold into the house and I knew that I would be saying goodbye to my best boy. He waited for us to be home together again. I tried to move him onto a dog bed and feed him, but he wasn't interested and all I could do was love him for the little time that I knew we had left together. Zara and Zoya took turns standing watch over him all that night as he laid in the hallway.

I wanted to lay with Z, but unfortunately, my condition would not let me lay on the floor with him, and I could not lift him onto the daybed, so I entrusted the night watch to the girls. I told him that I wasn't finished loving him, kissed him and went to sleep. A lifetime with him could never be enough! He passed in the night under the girls' watchful eye. Just as they kept watch over him, they also kept watch over me. Coming to check on me when they changed watch.

The next day, Mom helped me take his body to the crematorium. It had been horrific first night home, but I knew that this boy that was an angel on earth and in my life was going to forever be my guardian and would wait for me in heaven, just as he did on earth. The Rainbow Bridge gained a very special resident and my life would never be the same without him and would be forever changed because of him.

12.

SMILE!

I am not a fan of that request. I never have been and even more so now! It was a standard request or command from everyone that examined me. For me, it was a persistent reminder of yet another inadequacy. My smile was crooked. Plain and simply it sucked. Even when I laughed or was happy, I wasn't able to show it. I was going to look cross or angry in ever picture that was taken of me or I was going to show my stroke.

For someone that has been told that she always look grumpy or mad and that I need to smile more, this was one of the biggest kicks to the teeth. The faked smile was all that I had to change people's impression of me. Forcing a smile sucked already, but no being able to fake it was even worse. Now I couldn't even fake it!

The smile was a challenge that I WAS going to master! I was determined. My speech therapist

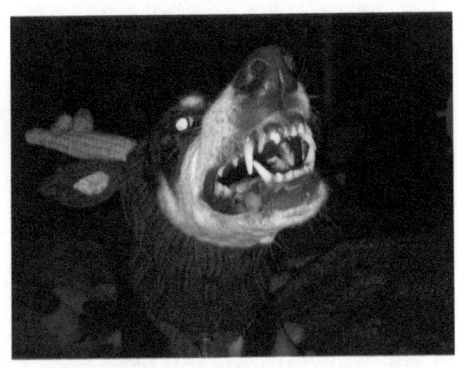

helped me a lot, by getting me to growl like my grumpy dog, Zollie. Jess made me growl every time I talked with her on FaceTime. All of the therapists were growled at when I said Hello. It was part of who I was to them. I would make them laugh, but they understood that it was helping me.

A few weeks after I was discharged, I was able to smile with some normalcy. It was crooked when I tried to smile, but it would come out naturally sometimes when I was genuinely happy. That was a huge accomplishment. It was

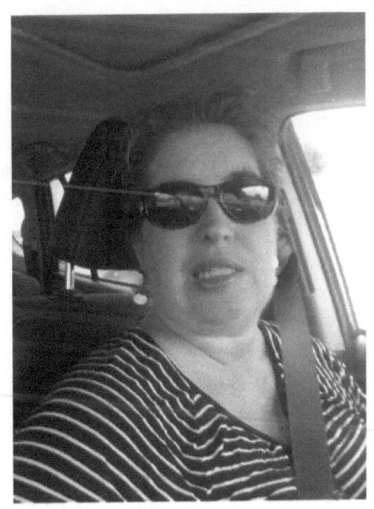

progress that people around me could see.

I still hate being told to smile, but I am happy that I can do it again.

There is still one little thing that is related to the smile, that bothers me and persists. I drool more when I sleep. It's not horrible, but it is noticeable to me. So, I have learned to sleep with my hand under my face/ mouth. I also can feel a build up of saliva when I am getting tired.

13.

Hi ho hi ho, It's back to work I Go!... or do I?

After several weeks of being home, visiting numerous doctors, and getting everyone's blessing, I was allowed to go back to work. My doctors were OK with me working without restrictions. They just told me to not push myself too hard and know when to rest. Work Pro agreed with my doctors and basically said that I should not be expected to walk long distances without assistance from a cart or vehicle.

Of course, when 'I got back, some people expected the old me and the ones that had visited me regularly when I was in the hospital and convalescing understood that I was different and were happy to just have me back. Their expectations were better, but no one else understood how real the struggles were.

I tripped and fell on an all weather entry rug one of my first days back. When the HR Director found out, I was told that I had to get approval from WorkPro for a second time to come back to work and until then, i was on Paid Administrative Leave. What the hell? I would have tripped on that rug without the stroke! I may not have fallen, but I would have tripped. I'm a klutz with a bad knee. It is the recipe for disaster.

I flew through the tests at Work Pro with no problems and they gave me full clearance, as did my primary care physician. I explained the trip to them and they all had a good laugh about it.The folks at work still wanted me on light duty, so they banned me from the events that I planned and even visits to summer camps and programs. Needless to say, I was pissed off about the way I was"handled". I was not able to make any of the overtime that I relied on from the events and was forced to watch other staff take over and take credit for the events that I spent years building. Vendors and contractors were calling and texting to tell me how much they missed me. They understood that it was not my decision, but, like me, they were not happy about the situation.

A few weeks after I went back for the second time, to be told that a co-worker complained about my attitude. Seriously? People really don't understand stroke recovery! Emotions become extremely heightened for many people, and I was no exception. After being drug through the wringer to even be allowed to go back to work, being told I couldn't do my job or earn the overtime that I relayed upon, now I have a bad attitude? Who wouldn't? Luckily, I love what I do and did not have the ability to quit on the spot, or I would have. I was pissed though. So, I put on my fake half smile and carried on, trying to have as little interaction with others in the office as possible. My office is located in the back of the department. So, I would take a deep breath when I got out of the car, put on the fake smile and "Good morning" my way back to my little cave, hoping that my boss wouldn't stop me to give me the laundry list of things that she wanted from me. I just wanted to make it until noon without being bombarded with things, so I could work through the list of things that I needed to do at my own pace and head to lunch feeling a sense of accomplishment, rather than being overwhelmed with stress and crying in my car for an hour.

14.

Goodbye Lockes

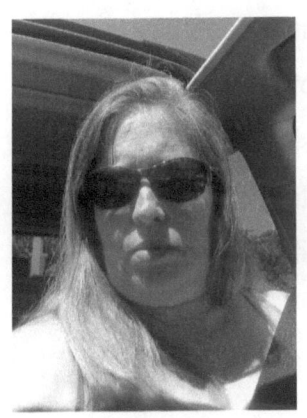 My hair was fairly long when I had the stroke. I typically let it grow out then cut it to shoulder length and then I get it cut and donate it. I've been doing it for years. I like to keep it long enough to put it in a ponytail or bun to keep it off my face and not so long that I look like a wanna be teenager, trying to hide from the world behind my hair.

When I had the stroke, I vomited quite a bit and it was all my hair because I was laying on my side and could not get up to go to the bathroom. At the hiospital, it wasn't washed for a week. I got it put up in a bun with help from my sister and daughter and it stayed that way until I made it to rehab, I had asked them to clean it in the first hospital, but that was not a priority for them, so the dried vomit and smell just became part of me. In rehab, they would help me wash my hair every few days and it was amazing, but I couldn't get it put up by myself, so I got some thick head bands to get it out of my face. I still hated it, So in the spring, after I got home and started back to work, , I finally quit! I got tired up unsuccessfully trying to put my hair up, so I got it all cut off. Much to the dismay of many, I opted to get the sides shaved down with a number 5 and a short, spiky top. It was a huge change and quite literally a weight lifted off of my shoulders.

I bought some really cool colored hair wax and spray and colored my hair to match my outfits. It was fun and I think it made my short hair a bit elegant. My favorite colors were the metallic ones: gold, silver and rose gold (a blend of red and gold wax).

The shock of my new do effected not, just me, but also those around me. One of my friend's was so shocked by the change, that he could not even look at me for more than 3 seconds. He hugged me, but kept his eyes down or to my side. It was quite bizarre and it still haunts me a little. I saw him again several

weeks ago and even though my hair has growing out, and I no longer color and spike it, he still has difficulty looking at me.

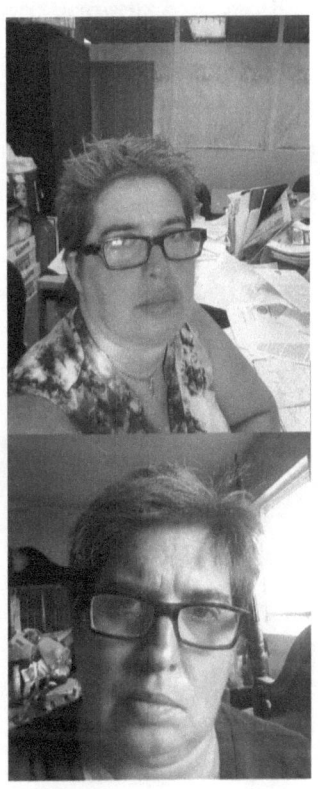

It got floppy on the top now and I hated it, but then decided to try another new do, so /I had the back cut and left the front longer., in sort of a Devil Wear Prada look (just not in silver). It's not bad. I can still wear headbands and hats, tuck it behind my ear, or style it back. I have

Not decided whether I will let it grow out or keep it short, but there are options that don't involve a bun out there, so I'm trying to keep an open mind about it. I don't need to look the way that I did for the last 20 years for the next 20.

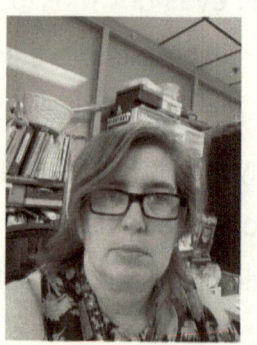

15.

PUPPIES!

There was a court date scheduled in May for the incident that happened on campus with my daughter. So, we packed our bags and started out for Tennessee. When we were halfway there, she got a call from her lawyer telling her that the hearing had been rescheduled for September. When she told me, all I could do was look at her and say, "Do you want to go to Georgia and look at some puppies?" So I called the rescue, we reprogrammed the GPS, and changed our hotel booking. We stayed overnight outside of Atlanta and met the people and puppies from the rescue the next morning. There were 2 boys left from the litter. Belgian Malnois Husky mixes. The combination had the potential to be great wheel dogs for my very muttly dogsled team. So, we looked at both puppies and number 2 stole my eyeglasses. I looked over at Jess, who was holding and cuddling number 4 and I said, "Zeek the Geek!" I switched puppies with her and looked at the piggy little face of number 4 and said, "Zazu". So, that was it. We were heading home with two new puppies. Balls of energy and sass, wrapped in fur.

Anyone that has ever had a puppy, know how much work they are. When you have two along with four other dogs, that increases at least three fold. The other dogs all start acting like the puppies, so, we knew we needed to start training and needed help with these crazy kids. I registered for a puppy class and Jess and I each had a dog to train. I had my little "Muffin Man", Zazu and Jess had Zeek the Geek. They did fine for the most part, but they were each other's squirrels.

My friend John, was one of the puppy class instructors. He was so helpful and sweet throughout the class. He would put screens up around the puppies so they would focus on the commands and not each other. He also always offered me a hand to get up when I was on the floor and with anything else that I needed. Again, I was grateful to have him as a friend and was so happy that he was helping with our class. I don't know if we puppies would have made it through without him.

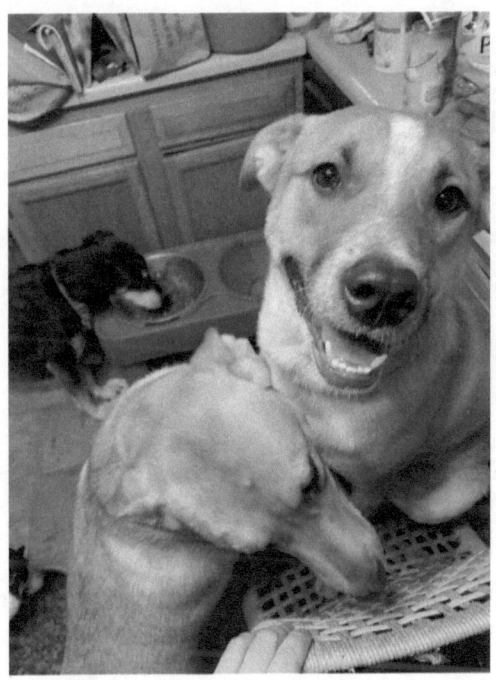

16.

PTSD

Most conversations about Post Traumatic Stress Disorder (PTSD) center around veterans returning from war or public safety officers that have seen or experienced horrific events that they keep reliving. Those are very real and difficult things to work through.

Stroke and other traumatic medical event survivors often have their own version of PTSD. This may cause panic attacks, difficulty sleeping or eating, and all around stress.

For me, it does exactly those things. I have panic attacks when I try to do household repairs alone. It has been over a year, and even though my sister and daughter got the Carper all out of my room, I have yet to finish the new floor. I break down every time I try to work on it. For me, it's an association with what I was doing when I had the stroke.

When I get a headache, I panic, but I'm also afraid to lay down with a headache. The same is true for feeling nauseous. I automatically start thinking it's a stroke and do things like tough my thumb to each finger to check my coordination.

There are other things that make me stress or panic, too. It could be a person, like the doctor that prescribed the medicine that caused the stroke, a day, or even just the thought of my daughter going back to school and being in the house alone.

I started seeing a psychotherapist about it and he taught me some very helpful acupressure techniques that can help calm me in a stressful situation. I appreciate learning the new techniques for relaxation without having to retell or relive the incident or focus on negativity as many therapists do. I go once a week and often just feel like I am in a better mental space when I leave his office. There was a week that was a bit awkward, so I needed to take a few weeks off to clear my own head. Sometimes you have to do that in order to get control of your life back. When I returned, he talked about cleaning up the mental and social clutter in my life. Funny, that is why I took the weeks off from therapy. He was distracting me from the things that I needed to focus on.

17.

V Day

I have a friend with benefits. On Valentines Day, just before the stroke, I was at a two day conference about two hours from home. I got a room at a local hotel so I wouldn't have a four hour drive each day. I had Hilton Honors points to cover the cost so staying there was the best thing to do. I have done the same thing other years and it's been nice. So rather than stay alone, I asked my friend to stay with me for the night. We don't see each other often and our benefits are not a regular thing (typically happen about once year). So, with the star alignment and the holiday, this was going to be a night with some benefits. We went out for dinner and then headed back to the room for dessert. We have been friends for many years, so pleasing each other comes very naturally. On this night, I was feeling especially satisfied and made the remark that I was going to have an aneurysm. That comment still haunts me. It was less than a week before the stroke and even the thought of intimacy still scares me over a year later. I know it didn't cause the stroke, but the foreshadowing is enough to terrify me.

The week of the next Valentines Day caused me I lot of anxiety. Not having a significant other brings anxiety of its own, but the thought of intimacy is now an extra stressor that I really didn't anticipate. The association with Valentines Day is even more bad juju during an already stressful time to be single.

18.

BERMUDA

I never thought a cruise to Bermuda would seem like a runner up trip, but that's what it was. After recovering to the point where I could walk comfortably with just a cane and do most things alone again, we booked a cruise to Bermuda. It could never replace SATS5, but made my feel slightly less guilty for making Jess miss it. I lived there for two and a half years in the early '90s and had only been there once since (when Jess was almost 3), so this was a chance for me to show her some of the places and things that I speak so fondly of on a regular basis. I took her to a local pub for a little drinking(which she was old enough to do there). we explored, we sat on the beach, and we had a great time on the ship, but it still was rather hollow. I proved to myself that I could be on a ship. I could walk, go to shows, etc. I needed that validation. It would never match SATS, but it was still a vacation. We were away from work, enjoying the company of one another, relaxing, and regrouping. I worked hard to increase my walking distances and stamina. I relaxed in a therapy pool for several days. I got stronger and it showed when I returned to physical therapy after the trip.

19.

The Healing Process

The healing process following a stroke is very different for everyone. For me, the biggest things in my favor were by age, fitness, desire, and determination. That last one is what most of my therapists will say made me different from many of their other patients. I was determined to do things on my own again.Little things like putting my hair in a ponytail and tying my shoes became challenges for me. Although I had my hair chopped off before I mastered the ponytail, that didn't stop me from trying a thousand times to do it. I braided it on the side a little and could do my daughter's hair, but the challenge of blindly doing the work behind my head was just more than I could mastering the time that I wanted. Giving up was not easy for me, but it was something that I needed to do and continue to to, because it is ok to know your limits and that was one of mine. I have no idea if I can do it yet because my hair is still too short to try.

Tying my shoes was a different story. I was determined to do master that, too. So, after my release, while I was living in my parent's living room, I tried it. I tried it every day and one day, after trying to do it a bit differently, Did it! I came up with a mostly one-handed tying technique that impressed my therapist, Mike. He told me that I should make a video to teach others how to do it. Perhaps I will!.my right hand does all of the work and Lucky(my left hand) just holds the pieces together. It's not something I would try to teach to a child, but for someone that already knows how to tie, it's a pretty easy modification. The key is using your index finger or middle to tuck the second loop through the hole at the end. Most days, I still wear slip on shoes, boots with zippers, or sandals, so I don't have to tie every day. But when I do wear sneakers that tie, it's no longer a stressful thing. I tie the laces fast and I'm on my way.

These seemingly little things are, not only great measuring tools for your progress, but also wonderful motivators. Once you master one thing, you can set another challenge.

Post stroke, one year, my sister was in town visiting my parents. I went to visit them all one day and she asked me if I could do a push-up. Well, that was one of my goals when I got out of the hospital, but I had yet to try. So, after my sister said that she did 5 the day before, I had to do 6. She sat there and watched in awe and we were all surprised that I could do one, never-the-less 6! And so the challenge began! I went to work the next day, determined to do one more than the day before. My work neighbor supervised and counted. 7! Yeah! Then 10, 12,15,20,25,30,35,50,60,and two weeks after I started, 75! Meanwhile, my sister was still doing about 40, which is a long way from her original 5, but wasn't quite to my number yet. I took a few days off, then did 100!! In two weeks, I went from 6 to 100. Granted, they were modified push ups, but they were still more than a lot of people can do, particularly a hear after a massive stroke.

These are the little victories that give you pride following so much defeat. So that's now the way that I look at my day. By victories! I give myself a point for everything I successfully do throughout the day. Some days I set a point goal. 10 points or wins a day seems to be a good number for me.

Did more pushups than I did yesterday -1 point

Loaded and ran the dishwasher-1 point

Finished 2 projects at work-2 points

Walked over a mile -1 point

Packed and ate what I packed for breakfast and lunch -2 points

.... and just like that, I'm at 8 points for the day.

So making dinner will add one and calling my parents on the drive home will add another and I have met my goal for the day. Easy Peasy! And if I don't get all of the points for the day, it's ok. Every point is one for something that I couldn't do at all a year ago, so it's a win even if I only get 1.other point achieving tasks are any work check list related items, going to yoga class or any other class or workshop where I can learn something new, social groups or outings with friends or family, grocery shopping, reading, writing, working in the house or yard. Whatever gives you the feeling of accomplishment, can be a point.

Some days, Got out of bed, Took a shower, and Got dressed is worthy of three points because mornings are even more difficult now than they used to be and I have never been a morning person and now, with limited energy, it is really a struggle some days. I'm glad they are pretty flexible with me at work. I text them when I'm running late and they understand. Typically its only 5 minutes, and I feel a sense of accomplishment if I am in before 9 a.m. (offices open at 8:30).It's not just my lack of morning motivation, but also trying to wrangle three dogs and a cat that thinks he's a dog in the morning, too. Zeek never wants to come in. He knows that it means going to his room (crate) and he always wants "5 more minutes" to play. He is a brat! Everyone else comes in, goes to their room and eats their breakfast, while I'm shaking the treat bag to get Zeek in the house. Once Zeek is in, everyone gets a treat, so they don't complain too much.

20.

Nashville Bound

The day for Jess' court date had come and there was no way she was going to do it alone. So, I hopped on a plane at 5 am and headed to Nashville. Jess met me at the airport and we went to court. We sat in front of her friend, who was also being accused, and his parents. The courtroom had nearly emptied before they were called before the judge. The lawyer was extremely nice and talked to the judge for her then he and her friend's lawyer went into a conference with the DA. Although the charges were not dropped, the fine was under $100 and minimal community service with expungement after 6 months, so the lawyers did a great job. Of course it didn't help that the accuser had no one in court with her... no friends or parents. It was such bullshit and I am still mad at the school official for calling Jess a liar when she was first accused and they were looking into the incident. Of course it was around the time of my stroke, so she was already stressed out.

I went to Tennessee several other times in the fall for football games, so I could seeJess in the marching band. Games were fun and I've become friends with several other band parents, so the tailgating became quite epic.

21.

DISNEY

Jess and I went to Disney a few weeks before my stroke. It was for my 48th birthday and happened to be over MLK weekend, which was also the Festival of The Arts at Epcot. We had an amazing time! It was a happy memory and I loved being able to remember the trip through the photos on my phone and iPad. Remembering the rides, the smells, and being able to do everything a "normal" person could do. I wanted to be that person again!

We had another trip to Disney planned for October for Jess's Birthday and I wanted it to be the same kind of experience.

I drove from Delaware to Orlando and slept briefly at rest stops on my way, then picked Jess up at the airport. We stayed one night at a hotel by the airport before moving closer to the parks.

I was determined to get back to being myself. With the exception of using a cane and getting tired faster, I was getting pretty close to my pre-stroke self for the trip in October. I rode the rides, stood in line, and loved every second of the time that I was able to spend with my daughter. This was proof to myself that I was OK!

Our hotel was prefect, with a large soaking tub and a great view of the Magic Kingdom from the balcony where we could sit and watch the fireworks at night, after leaving the parks early to keep my exhaustion at bay. This was an unexpected bonus for the trip and was greatly appreciated.

Our first stop on the first day was Muppetvision 3D and my daughter bought me a great Fozzy Bear hat that became my go to hat for the week. It was fun and whimsical and suited me

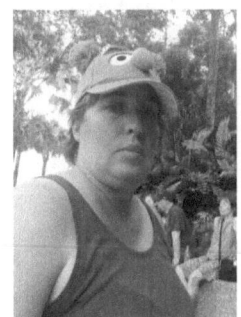

perfectly. It was a happy hat! Wokka Wokka!

The day that we spent at Epcot was beautiful, but since we knew the park would require covering a lot of ground, I rented a scooter for the day. Aside from the high cost, it was perfect. I zipped around and did not feel like a burden that day Getting the scooter was a very difficult thing for me, but it was a good decision and I'm glad I did it. I probably should have done it at Animal Kingdom and the Magic Kingdom, too, but I was proving my abilities to myself. I worked hard to get to this point and needed to do it. I also wanted my daughter to see that I was alright and that we could still do adventurous things together.

The biggest excitement for me was riding the new Slinky Dog Dash rollercoaster and visiting Toy Story Land.

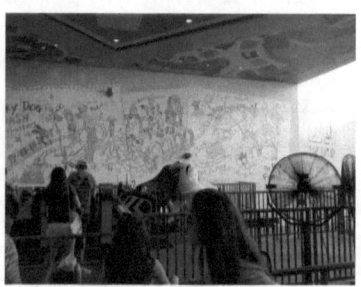

Of course, I took a lot longer to do many things and she was very patient with me, giving me the spot by the rail in ride queues, picking up food from the counters and letting me sit and wait. This trip was a bit slower paced than what we typically have, but there was not one complaint or frustration from her. She was genuinely grateful to be there with me and happy that I was able to do as much as I could. I was the only one that was frustrated at my pace and energy level.

We watched the fireworks from the hotel, rather than the parks and didn't stay until closing every night, so I could get extra sleep. They were pretty small concessions, really, but made a huge impact on my ability to function each day.

Taking a slower pace was quite difficult for me because I have not typically been one to take things slow.so it was quite a challenge. More so for me than Jess, because she has the patience of Job from spending time with her grandparents and working at summer camps. Plus, she was happy to have me alive and able to do things with her, so she was grateful and showed it.

22.

FALLING or FAILING; IT FEELS THE SAME

So, here I am, over a year post stroke, and I fell yesterday and again today. Yesterday was a nice, graceful slip in the grass that ended in a split of sorts, when I was walking in the grass to my car. I lightly hit my knee and the top of one shoe got wet, but that was it. No witnesses. No embarrassment. No need to change or readjust. Just get up, brush off, and move on. It was that simple.

Today's fall was far worse. Walking into the office, a bit late, as usual, trying to carry my work bag, lunch bag, water cup and coffee mug. I tripped on a rubber mat. My shoe caught on the rubber and as usual, my very weak ankle gave way and down I went. There was a customer in the lobby next to where I fell who very nicely asked if I needed help or was ok. I told him that I was fine, but the ladies in finance went off on there typical over reaction and were screaming that I fell all over the first floor. So, the Calvary came running! People were grabbing my bags, cups, putting their hands out, etc. Really guys... I'm OK. I twisted my ankle and fell. I've done it many times. The customer that saw it, had picked up my water and coffee and turn to everyone and said, "She must be an expert at falling! She didn't even spill her coffee! Damn straight!

Yes, it's true. Especially since the stroke, I've fallen at least 5 or 6 times at work and probably close to the same at home. Luckily, I haven't been hurt, and there have been some other close calls, but every time, I fall, it takes me back to the first few days back to work, when I fell and they put me on light duty and sent me through the gauntlet of doctors' approvals that I really could be back at work. I have had bad ankles since I was doing gymnastics in elementary school and I am a bit of a klutz. It's a bad combination that means that when I catch my now slow to respond foot on anything, my ankle is going to give out and I'm going down!

Top all of that off with two bad knees and sciatica and it's the perfect combination of critical failure of the stroke effected leg. I'm doomed to fall. Over and over again until there is a doctor that will fix something, rather than mask it!

23.

IN THE BEGINNING

My bad knees and fat ass are what started this whole thing to begin with. I need partial knee replacements, but they wouldn't consider doing them with my weight at 250. They needed me to get and stay under 200 to do the partial replacement. My endocrinologist said that the med that had helped me lose weight before could help, so, even though I told him on several occasions that it made my blood pressure high, he gave it to me again to use as I needed it. That medication that made my blood pressure high, caused the stroke. It's been a very vicious circle with no end in sight. I've lost 50 pounds since I got home from the hospital, but 20 to 30 occasionally finds its way to my butt.

Exercise is great, unless you have bad joints that don't let you bear weight. I was a personal trainer and once helped the crew of a ship lose 2 tons of body fat while they were on a 6 month deployment. Every summer, I lose almost 25 pounds just because I have a garden with lots of fresh veggies for salads and soups and I walk a lot (when I can).

The pressure and stress of losing weight in order to get a needed medical procedure, so you can exercise and feel better is crazy! I know plenty of people over 200 pounds that had full knee replacements without any problems.why is that not an option for me? I hear things like, "you're too young", and, "wait a few years" with many physical repairs or fixes. Really? Do you let the bad tires on your car go because it's only 2 years old? Or do you find the best ones out there and get them replaced and run the crap out of them?

They said it about a neck fusion I had 15 years ago. My response was that I wanted to try to have normalcy back and if it didn't work, fine, but I needed to try. I feel the same way about my knees. I want to walk without feeling like I'm on the verge of falling or walk up stairs with out holding only the handrails for dear life. I want to run with my grandchildren some day and teach them how to play soccer. Right now, I can't envision that.

I want to eventually have a wellness and arts farm, with gardens, animals, and arts centers. I need to be able to keep up with that. The way that my knees currently are, that will not be possible.

The physical ailments do as much or more damage to the mind than they do the body sometimes. Just as my falls are failures in my mind, so are all of my inabilities. The short comings are failures. Incompetences of the body preclude those of the mind. It's hard to think about managing a nursery and greenhouses when you fear walking on the uneven ground and know that you will be in pain daily.

Here is where I am throwing in a suggestion for the medical teams of stroke patients; While patients are in the hospital or rehab, consider the pre-existing conditions or even new conditions that may need to be treated while they are in a place that can help fix them. Bring in orthopedic specialists, massage therapists, chiropractors, eye doctors, etc. that can help the patient truly get back to where they would like to be. It may not be pre-stroke. It may be better. If you know that they have a bad knee and there has been talk of replacement, bring those doctors in as part of the care team, too. They may be able to help the patient find more success by providing an injection or surgery that can relieve pain, expand flexibility, and thereby improve mental well being and motivation. Bracing a weak body part, getting an MRI to find the cause of pain or weakness can be an important part of recovery. Understand that pain relief is part physical and part mental and that not all short fillings are because of a stroke. Deficiencies exist pre-stroke that may affect recovery.

I'm not saying that my care team ignored the pre-existing condition of my knees, but they did not seek out tests to confirm or any specific care for it. They happily helped me put a brace on and left it at that.

24.

PLEASURES

One of my small pleasures in daily life, is a bath. I love bubble baths, hot tubs, saunas....Places where I can warm my muscles and revive my spirit with scents and sensations. The warmth, particularly in winter, is spiritually uplifting. It helps me find inner peace and center myself. I like to add dish soap and essential oils to my bath. Lavender helps me relax when I've had a rough day and dish soap bubbles seem to last longer than traditional bubble bath. If it's good and gentle enough to clean oily penguins, it's good enough for me!

I believe that Stroke,as well as, other recovering patients need to have some of their typical pleasures. A bath, a favorite meal, cozy pajamas, fuzzy slippers. Comfort is key! Believe me, the weeks and months of discomfort and confusion are overwhelming, so any comfort that can be provided is absolutely welcomed! Personally, while I was in rehab, I looked forward to shower days with Thelma, my aid and friend of the family. She gave the best scalp massages when she shampooed my hair. It was the most relaxation I got while I was in rehab. It sounds like a simple thing, and I suppose it is, but she cared and took her time, rubbing my neck as well as the scalp. I am grateful for her friendship and care that she provided my father during his stays on the rehab floor and for the care that she provided to me. She is one of those saints in scrubs that I have referenced.My family and friends helped with providing me with comforts like favorite foods, cookies, comfortable clothes and shoes. A warm fluffy blanket would have been nice, but the heated ones at the hospital were adequate, but not super cozy or comforting. Decent headphones are also a huge plus. The cheap institutional ones just don't do the job for listening to music or tv..

25.

RIDING THE WAVE

It is hard for me to think too far or clearly about the future now. Life's thrown a lot of curveballs in the past two years so, althoughI have dreams and desires, I am trying not to get too far ahead of myself.

Besides the ups and downs, of which, I have already written, I had another very traumatic incident a few weeks ago. My puppy, Zazu, died unexpectedly after eating a cassette tape. It's affect on me was far worse than I ever could have predicted. I was, and still am, overcome with grief. He had the sweetest soul, like Zenith, and I miss him terribly. He died by my side and with his brother next to him, so I know he went knowing he was loved, but that doesn't help the feeling of helplessness and sadness.

I had therapy in the afternoon after Zazu died. It was the most awful and awkward session to date. The therapist didn't know what to say and I left feeling worse than when I went in.

I took several weeks off following that session because I needed to be the voice in my own head for a while. I needed to cry my eyes out over my lost baby. He was only a year old and had not even been with me a year.

His brother, Zeek, was as sad and los as I, so we found comfort in each other. The day after his death, We had a Mommy-Zeeky day. We went to visit my office, got ice cream (which he threw up in the car), and went to visit Grandma and PopPop, who, of course made a big fuss over him. We both came home feeling better and a little more bonded.

Jess never called after I texted her about Zazu. She's all grown up and pushing away in order to gain her independence. It's hard for me because we have always been very close and now sometimes it's weeks between her calls and when she's home, she doesn't really want to hang out with me anymore,

I think this is one of the circumstances where the stroke effect applies and intensifies the pain and disappointment. The feeling of being an outcast and possibly undeserving of the second chance that I got.

About The Author

Sharon Watt has over 30 years of experience as a recreation professional with both the military (Navy) and local government agencies. She considers herself an adventurer with an adult daughter and a myriad of four legged children. In her free time, she enjoys crafting, home improvements, mushing, and gardening.

In 2018, Sharon endured a massive, life-changing, hemmoragic stroke that nearly took her life. With hard work and determination, she has recovered. She began writing following the stroke as therapy to return to work as a community event planner. Then decided that her story is worth sharing and wrote her first book, Strokus.

Sharon is proving that brain trauma can be a stepping stone to the future, an adjustment to life's path, and a motivation to those around the afflicted

Although she has been in the field of recreation for decades, she has always loved writing and has served as the playbill editor in high school, the Delaware Recreation and Parks Society's Newsletter editor, and has written many articles and news releases to promote her department's programs and events throughout her career. Her matter-of-fact style will entertain readers while giving facts, telling stories, and teaching lessons.